Table of Contents

INTRODUCTION 12

WHAT IS A DYSPHAGIA SOFT DIET? 13

WHY A DYSPHAGIA DIET IS NEEDED 14

LEVELS OF A DYSPHAGIA DIET 15

PREPARING FOOD AND LIqUIDS 17

CHECKING YOUR HEALTH 18

GETTING ENOUGH LIqUIDS 19

WHEN TO CALL YOUR HEALTHCARE PROVIDER ... 20

VEGETABLES AND FRUITS 21

Foods to choose: 21

Foods to avoid: 21

GRAIN FOODS 22

Foods to choose: 22

Foods to avoid: 23

PROTEIN FOODS 23

Foods to choose: 23

Foods to avoid: 25

DESSERTS AND SNACKS 26

Foods to choose: 26

Foods to avoid: 26

WHO NEEDS A SOFT FOOD DIET? 26

DYSPHAGIA SOFT DIET RECIPIES 27

    TURKEY AND DUMPLING SOUP............................. 27

        INGREDIENTS.. 27

        DIRECTIONS 28

    MACARONI AND CHEESE 28

        INGREDIENTS.. 28

        DIRECTIONS 29

    COLD-DAY CHICKEN NOODLE SOUP 30

        INGREDIENTS.. 30

        DIRECTIONS 30

    MASHED POTATOES WITH CHEDDAR...................... 31

        INGREDIENTS.. 31

        DIRECTIONS 31

    CHOCOLATE AVOCADO PUDDING 31

        INGREDIENTS.. 31

        DIRECTIONS 32

    APPLE CRUMBLE... 32

        INGREDIENTS.. 32

        DIRECTIONS 32

    BAKED CUSTARD... 33

        INGREDIENTS.. 33

        DIRECTIONS 33

    MAPLE SWEET CARROT PUREE 34

INGREDIENTS 34

INSTRUCTIONS 34

PUMPKIN BROWNIE PUREE 35

Ingredients: 35

INSTRUCTIONS: 35

MEAT LOAF PUREE 36

INGREDIENTS: 36

INSTRUCTIONS: 36

CRUSHED ICE (IN A BLENDER) 36

INGREDIENTS 37

INSTRUCTIONS 37

ORANGE FRAPPE 37

INGREDIENTS 37

INSTRUCTIONS 37

COTTAGE CHEESE COCKTAIL 38

INGREDIENTS 38

INSTRUCTION 38

FRUIT DRINK 38

INGREDIENTS 38

INSTRUCTIONS 38

STRAWBERRY NECTAR 39

INGREDIENTS 39

INSTRUCTIONS 39

VIRGIN PINA COLADA 40

INGREDIENTS... 40

    INSTRUCTIONS... 40

CHOCOLATE BANANA MALT 40

INGREDIENTS... 40

    INSTRUCTIONS... 41

CUSTARD NOG... 41

INGREDIENT 41

    INSTRUCTIONS... 41

CREAMY MILKSHAKE.. 41

INGREDIENTS... 41

    INSTRUCTIONS... 42

EXTRA THICK MILKSHAKE 42

INGREDIENTS... 42

    INSTRUCTIONS... 42

SPECIAL "INSTANT BREAKFAST" SHAKE.................. 42

INGREDIENTS... 42

STRAWBERRYEBANANA MILKSHAKE 43

INGREDIENTS... 43

CHILLED GLASSES... 43

INGREDIENTS... 43

APRICOT SMOOTHIE 44

INGREDIENTS... 44

BANANA SMOOTHIE 44

INGREDIENTS.. 44

COFFEE SMOOTHIE 45

INGREDIENTS.. 45

DREAMSICLE SMOOTHIE 45

INGREDIENTS.. 45

MELON SMOOTHIE 46

INGREDIENTS.. 46

MINTED MELON SMOOTHIE 46

INGREDIENTS.. 46

PEACH SMOOTHIE 47

INGREDIENTS.. 47

PINEAPPLE SMOOTHIE 47

YOGURT STRAWBERRY SMOOTHIE 48

INGREDIENTS.. 48

LEMON CHEESE CAKE 48

INGREDIENTS.. 48

TOPPING... 49

INGREDIENTS.. 49

LEMONY LIGHT CHEESE CAKE 49

INGREDIENTS.. 49

APPLE CUSTARD 50

INGREDIENTS.. 50

BAKED CARAMEL CUSTARD 51

INGREDIENTS... 51

COTTAGE CHEESE CUSTARD................................... 52

INGREDIENTS... 52

EGG CUSTARD 52

INGREDIENTS... 52

PINEAPPLE RICE CUSTARD 53

INGREDIENTS... 53

PUMPKIN CUSTARD 54

INGREDIENTS... 54

LIME DIVINE 55

INGREDIENTS... 55

LIME-PEAR DESSERT 56

INGREDIENTS... 56

APRICOT CHIFFON PIE.. 56

INGREDIENTS... 56

CHEESECAKE PIE 58

INGREDIENTS... 58

CHOCOLATE CHIFFON PIE 58

INGREDIENTS... 58

FROZEN CRANBERRY VELVET PIE............................ 59

INGREDIENTS... 59

EGG NOG PIE 60

INGREDIENTS... 60

IMPOSSIBLE PIE 61

INGREDIENTS... 61

KEY LIME PIE 61

VEGETABLES 63

CONGEALED AVOCADO SALAD 63

INGREDIENTS... 63

BAKED BEANS 63

MEXICAN REFRIED BEANS 64

INGREDIENTS... 64

SWEDISH BAKED BEANS..................................... 64

INGREDIENTS... 64

CARROT CUSTARD 65

INGREDIENTS... 65

CARROT ORANGE PURBE 66

INGREDIENTS... 66

CARROT PUDDING 67

INGREDIENTS... 67

BROWN SAUCE FOR CARROT PUDDING 68

INGREDIENTS... 68

CARROTS WITH A TWIST 69

EGGPLANT CASSEROLE 69

INGREDIENTS... 69

PUR~ED PEAS 70

INGREDIENTS.. 70

GRATED POTATO CASSEROLE.................................. 71

INGREDIENTS.. 71

POTATO GOURMET 72

INGREDIENTS.. 72

POTATO NESTS 72

BAKED SWEET POTATOES 73

BLENDED SWEET POTATOES 73

INGREDIENTS.. 73

MASHED SWEET POTATOES 73

SWEET POTATO SOUFFL~....................................... 74

INGREDIENTS.. 74

RICOTTA SPINACH BAKE... 75

INGREDIENTS.. 75

SPINACH SOUFFLE 76

INGREDIENTS.. 76

CRAB BISQUE... 77

INGREDIENTS.. 77

CURRIED FISH BISQUE.. 78

INGREDIENTS.. 78

LOBSTER BISQUE 78

INGREDIENTS.. 78

SALMON BISQUE 79

INGREDIENTS... 79

BASIC SEAFOOD BISQUE 80

INGREDIENTS... 80

SHRIMP BISQUE c COLD 81

INGREDIENTS... 81

TUNA CHOWDER 81

INGREDIENTS... 81

CHICKEN AVOCADO SOUP COLD 82

INGREDIENTS... 82

CHICKEN BISQUE 82

INGREDIENTS... 82

CURRIED CHICKEN SOUP......................... 83

INGREDIENTS... 83

YOGURT BORSCHT COLD......................... 84

INGREDIENTS... 84

BROCCOLI CHOWDER 84

INGREDIENTS... 84

CARROT VICHYSSOISE COLD.................... 85

INGREDIENTS... 85

CAULIFLOWER SOUP.............................. 86

INGREDIENTS... 86

THICKENED STRAINED CREAM SOUP....................... 87

INGREDIENTS... 87

CUCUMBER VICHYSSOISE COLD 87

INGREDIENTS... 87

CURRIED LEEK SOUP COLD..................................... 88

INGREDIENTS... 88

CREAM OF MUSHROOM SOUP 89

INGREDIENTS... 89

MUSHROOM VELVET SOUP..................................... 89

INGREDIENTS... 89

VICHYSSOISE ORIENTAL COLD 90

INGREDIENTS... 90

FRESH PEA SOUP 91

INGREDIENTS... 91

GREEN POTAGE 92

INGREDIENTS... 92

CREAM OF POTATO SOUP...................................... 93

INGREDIENTS... 93

SWEET POTATO SOUP.. 94

INGREDIENTS... 94

VEGETABLE BISQUE 95

INGREDIENTS... 95

BASIC CREAM OF VEGETABLE SOUP 95

INGREDIENTS... 95

PERFECTION VEGETABLE SOUP 96

INGREDIENTS... 96

VEGETABLE VICHYSSOISE COLD............................. 97

INGREDIENTS... 97

SAUCES 98

ALFREDO SAUCE.. 98

INGREDIENTS... 98

HERBED LEMON BUTTER SAUCE 99

INGREDIENTS... 99

MUSHROOM BUTTER SAUCE 99

INGREDIENTS... 99

QUICK HERBED HOLLANDAISE SAUCE 100

INGREDIENTS.. 100

ZESTY SALMON SAUCE.................................... 100

INGREDIENTS.. 100

CONCLUTION... 101

INTRODUCTION

A dysphagia diet is a special eating plan. Your healthcare provider may advise it if you have trouble swallowing (dysphagia).

Problems with swallowing can occur at any time and may not be known to that person or caregivers. It is important to be aware of swallowing difficulties due to the high occurrence of choking and aspiration associated with them. There are clues that can help identify when someone is having swallowing difficulties, however, many people can also have what is known as "silent aspiration". Many factors can compromise someone's ability to swallow safely. These are outlined below. Aging may be enough to compromise someone's swallowing abilities but the addition of medications may make this much worse. Medications such as those used for allergies or urinary incontinence cause a dry mouth making swallowing more difficult. Antipsychotic medications can cause both a dry mouth and affect the muscles of the face and tongue which are involved in swallowing. Medications that depress the central nervous system can decrease awareness and voluntary muscle control that may affect swallowing. These include medications used to treat seizures, antianxiety drugs, narcotics and muscle relaxants. The following information may seem very technical at times but it is important for understanding all the problems that can occur. This paper includes information regarding diets that may be ordered by a swallowing specialist or medical provider or that should be considered based on a person's age, medications, medical problems, and physical abilities even if that person hasn't had a formal swallowing evaluation.

WHAT IS A DYSPHAGIA SOFT DIET?

A dysphagia soft diet is needed if you have trouble chewing or swallowing. This can happen for many reasons such as mouth pain, poorly-fitting dentures, or missing teeth. Children going through tooth development may also have difficulties chewing or swallowing.

On a dysphagia soft diet you may eat foods that are soft and moist. Add broth, melted butter or soft margarine, gravy, sauces, milk, or juice to your foods for extra moisture.

Foods that are not soft or moist enough may need to be diced, minced, finely shaved, or mashed.

Foods that need to be diced should be cut into pieces that are smaller than 1 cm (about ½ inch) for adults and smaller than 8 mm for children.

WHY A DYSPHAGIA DIET IS NEEDED

When you have dysphagia, you are at risk for aspiration. Aspiration is when food or liquid enters the lungs by accident. It can cause pneumonia and other problems. The foods you eat can affect your ability to swallow. For example, soft foods are easier to swallow than hard foods. A dysphagia diet can help prevent aspiration. You may be at risk for aspiration from dysphagia if you have any of these medical conditions:

- Stroke
- Severe dental problems
- Conditions that lead to less saliva, such as

14

Sjogren syndrome
- Mouth sores
- Parkinson disease or other neurologic conditions
- Muscular dystrophies
- Blockage in the esophagus, such as a growth from cancer
- History of radiation therapy or surgery for throat cancer

You may need to follow a dysphagia diet for only a short time. Or you may be on it for a while. It depends on what is causing your dysphagia and how serious it is. A speech-language pathologist (SLP) assesses a person with dysphagia. The SLP will determine your risk for aspiration and talk about the best food and drink choices for you.

LEVELS OF A DYSPHAGIA DIET

The Academy of Nutrition and Dietetics has created a diet plan for people with dysphagia. The plan is called the National Dysphagia Diet. The dysphagia diet has 4 levels of foods. The levels are:

- Level 1. These are foods that are pureed

or smooth, like pudding. They need no chewing. This includes foods such as yogurt, mashed potatoes with gravy to moisten it, smooth soups, and pureed vegetables and meats.

- Level 2. These are moist foods that need some chewing. They include soft, cooked, or mashed fruits or vegetables, soft or ground meats moist with gravy, cottage cheese, peanut butter, and soft scrambled eggs. You should avoid crackers, nuts, and other dry foods.

- Level 3. This includes soft-solid foods that need more chewing. This includes meat, fruit, and vegetables that are easy to cut or mash. You should avoid crunchy, sticky, or very dry foods. This includes nuts, crackers, chips, and other snack foods.

- Level 4. This level includes all foods.

- You will also need to be careful about the liquids you drink. Talk with your SLP about the liquids that are allowed on your dysphagia diet. Here is more information on managing liquids in a dysphagia diet.

PREPARING FOOD AND LIQUIDS

Your SLP will give you instructions about how to prepare your food. You may need to avoid certain foods, or make changes to some foods. For example, you may need to puree your food. Make sure to taste and season your food before pureeing it. It will be easier to adjust to a new diet if your food smells and tastes appealing.

You may also need to make liquids thicker. You can manage your liquids by making thin liquids thicker. This is done by adding a flavorless gel, gum, powder, or other liquid to it. These are called thickeners. You can also buy pre-thickened liquids. Talk with your SLP if you have any questions about managing your liquids.

While you eat

While eating or drinking, it may help to sit upright, with your back straight. You may need support pillows to get into the best position. It may also help to have few distractions while eating or drinking. Changing between solid food and liquids may also help your swallowing. Stay upright for at least 30 minutes after eating. This can help reduce the risk for aspiration.

Watch for symptoms of aspiration such as:

- Coughing or wheezing during or right after eating
- Excess saliva
- Shortness of breath or fatigue while eating
- A wet-sounding voice during or after eating or drinking
- Fever 30 to 60 minutes after eating

After you eat

After meals, it's important to do proper oral care. The SLP can give you instructions for your teeth or dentures. Make sure to not swallow any water during your oral care routine.

CHECKING YOUR HEALTH

Your healthcare team will keep track of how well you are swallowing. You may need follow-up tests such as a fiberoptic endoscopic evaluation of swallowing (FEES) test. If your swallowing gets better or worse, your SLP may change your dysphagia diet over time. In time you may be able to eat and drink foods and liquids of all kinds.

While on a dysphagia diet, you may have trouble taking in enough fluid. This can cause dehydration, which can lead to serious health problems. Talk with your healthcare team about how you can help prevent this. In some cases drinking thicker liquids may make some of your medicines work less well. Because of this, you may need some of your medicines changed for a while.

While you are on a dysphagia diet

- Follow all instructions about what food and drink you can have.
- Do swallowing exercises as advised.
- Do not change your food or liquids, even if your swallowing gets better. Talk with your health care provider first.
- Crush medicines and mix them with food as needed.
- Tell all healthcare providers and caregivers that you are on a dysphagia diet. Explain which foods and liquids you can and cannot have.

Call 911

Call 911 if you have trouble breathing because of food blocking your airway.

WHEN TO CALL YOUR HEALTHCARE PROVIDER

Call your healthcare provider right away if you have any of these:

- Trouble swallowing that gets worse
- Unplanned weight loss
- Chewed food coming back up into the mouth
- Vomiting

Eating well

Canada's Food Guide recommends eating a variety of healthy foods each day. This includes:

- Having plenty of vegetables and fruits
- Choosing whole grain foods
- Eating protein foods

VEGETABLES AND FRUITS

Foods to choose:

- soft diced cooked vegetables (carrots, squash), mashable cooked vegetables (peas, spinach) or minced cooked vegetables (broccoli, yellow or green beans)
- very finely shredded or minced salads (coleslaw, leafy greens, lettuce) with extra dressing if needed
- mashed potatoes or other well-cooked potato side dishes such as scalloped potatoes
- canned cream corn
- soft ripe mashable fruit: canned, fresh, or frozen (bananas, canned crushed pineapple, canned mandarin oranges, canned sliced peaches, ripe pears), fresh fruit with skins and membranes removed (diced soft cantaloupe, seedless watermelon) fruit cocktail without pineapple pieces or grapes
- pureed, stewed pitted prunes
- fruit smoothies

Foods to avoid:

- hard, raw vegetables that cannot be mashed (broccoli, carrot sticks, cauliflower, celery), even if diced

- tossed salad, or any other salads made with ingredients not allowed
- salad or cabbage that is not finely shredded (Caesar, spinach, tossed)
- crispy dry French fries, hash browns, or potato skins
- whole kernel corn, even in soup
- fresh or canned vegetables or fruits, with membranes or tough skins (whole apples, citrus fruits, grapes, whole tomatoes)
- fruits with hard seeds (blackberries, raspberries)
- dried fruit (coconut, cranberries, raisins)
- pineapple, fresh or canned, sliced, chunks, or tidbits

GRAIN FOODS

Foods to choose:

- cooked cereals (cream of rice, Cream of Wheat® oat bran, oatmeal)
- cold cereals that soften in milk (bran flakes, corn flakes, rice crisps)
- soft moist bread products (biscuits, buns, buttered toast, muffins) served with butter, soft margarine, or other allowed spreads
- French toast, pancakes, or waffles, served

with applesauce or syrup to moisten
- soft moist barley, couscous, quinoa, or rice in sauces, soups, or casseroles
- pasta served in sauce
- bread pudding, or soft and moist bread stuffing (without chocolate chips, coconut, dried fruit, nuts, seeds, or any other hard particles)
- soft crackers, such as soda crackers
- soft cereal bars, such as Nutri-Grain® bars
- ground flax seed or wheat bran stirred into cereals

Foods to avoid:

- cereals or grain products (with chocolate chips, coconut, dried fruit, nuts, or seeds)
- dry, crusty, or chewy breads (bagels, crusty buns, English muffins, pitas, tortillas)
- dry, loose rice (brown, fried, steamed, wild)
- hard or chewy cereal bars, crackers, or granola
- dry pizza crust, such as thin crust pizza

PROTEIN FOODS

Foods to choose:

- milk: plain or flavoured
- buttermilk, smooth milkshakes, or fortified soy beverages
- smooth yogurt or fruit yogurt with small soft pieces of fruit
- cottage cheese
- all cheeses (hard or soft), diced, sliced, or grated
- soft tofu/soy protein
- soft cooked beans, lentils, peas, or soft dishes made with allowed ingredients (soft bean salad)
- smooth nut butters mixed into allowed foods (peanut butter smoothie)
- all cooked eggs or egg substitutes including omelets and quiche, made with allowed foods
- soft moist tender meat or poultry, diced
- canned fish with bones removed (canned salmon with mashed bones is allowed)
- tender boneless fish that flakes easily
- thinly shaved soft deli meats (roast beef, turkey, ham)
- sandwiches with finely-minced salad-type fillings (egg, chicken, tuna salad, minced lettuce, or cheese) without whole lettuce or whole raw vegetables
- tender mashable meats, made with allowed ingredients (casseroles, chili, lasagna,

meatloaf, meatballs, shepherd's pie, or stew)

- soft and mashable perogies, served with allowed condiments
- stir-fry made with allowed ingredients
- spaghetti sauces made with allowed ingredients
- broth or cream soups made with allowed ingredients

Foods to avoid:

- yogurt (with large fruit pieces, dried fruit, nuts, seeds, or granola)
- crispy melted stringy cheese topping (for example, on top of casserole)
- nut butters: crunchy or smooth, spread on food
- nuts and seeds, whole or chopped
- hard fried eggs
- bacon, bacon bits, or beef jerky
- crispy or dry fish, meat, or poultry
- casseroles, chili, or stews, made with ingredients not allowed
- processed luncheon meats, sausages, or wieners with hard casings such as garlic sausage, Kolbassa, or salami
- hamburgers or wieners in a bun

DESSERTS AND SNACKS

Foods to choose:

- ice cream, Popsicles®, sherbet, soy frozen desserts, or frozen yogurt
- smooth custards, milk pudding, mousse, rice pudding, or tapioca pudding
- soft, moist, or easy-to-break cookies (digestive biscuits)
- soft baked desserts (cream or pumpkin pies, moist cakes) made with allowed foods
- jellied desserts

Foods to avoid:

- baked desserts, custards, or puddings with chocolate chips, dried fruit, nuts, or seeds
- crispy or hard dry desserts and snacks
- chips, nachos, popcorn, or pretzels
- hard candy, gum, licorice, or toffee

WHO NEEDS A SOFT FOOD DIET?

Soft food diets are usually prescribed by healthcare practitioners to post-surgery patients and people with certain medical conditions.

Soft food diets are common in hospitals, long-term care facilities, and even at home. Usually, soft food diets have to be followed for short periods of a few days to a few weeks. But in some circumstances the diet may need to be followed for a longer period or for patients with dysphagia, a soft food diet will become their only option.

DYSPHAGIA SOFT DIET RECIPIES

TURKEY AND DUMPLING SOUP

INGREDIENTS

- 1 tablespoon olive oil
- 2 celery ribs, chopped
- 1/2 cup chopped onion
- 1-1/2 pounds red potatoes (about 5 medium), cut into 1/2-inch cubes
- 3-1/2 cups frozen mixed vegetables (about 16 ounces)
- 1/2 teaspoon pepper
- 1/2 teaspoon dried thyme
- 2 cartons (32 ounces each) reduced-sodium chicken broth
- 2-1/2 cups coarsely shredded cooked

turkey or chicken
- 2 cups biscuit/baking mix
- 2/3 cup 2% milk

• In a 6-qt. stockpot, heat oil over medium heat; saute celery and onion until tender, 3-4 minutes. Stir in potatoes, mixed vegetables, seasonings and broth; bring to a boil. Reduce heat; cook, covered, until potatoes are almost tender, 8-10 minutes. Add turkey; bring mixture to a simmer.

• Meanwhile, stir baking mix and milk until a soft dough forms; drop by tablespoonfuls on top of simmering soup. Cook, covered, on low heat until a toothpick inserted in dumplings comes out clean, 8-10 minutes.

MACARONI AND CHEESE

INGREDIENTS

- 1-1/2 cups uncooked elbow macaroni
- 5 tablespoons butter, divided
- 3 tablespoons all-purpose flour
- 1/2 teaspoon salt

- 1/4 teaspoon pepper
- 1-1/2 cups whole milk
- 1 cup shredded cheddar cheese
- 2 ounces cubed cheese
- 2 tablespoons dry bread crumbs

DIRECTIONS

• Cook macaroni according to package directions. Meanwhile, in a saucepan, melt 4 tablespoons of butter over medium heat. Stir in flour, salt and pepper until smooth. Gradually add milk. Bring to a boil; cook and stir for 2 minutes or until thickened. Reduce heat. Add the cheeses, stirring until the cheese is melted. Drain macaroni.

• Transfer macaroni to a greased 1-1/2-qt. baking dish. Pour cheese sauce over macaroni; mix well. Melt the remaining butter; add the breadcrumbs. Sprinkle over top. Bake, uncovered, at 375° for 30 minutes or until heated through and topping is golden brown

COLD-DAY CHICKEN NOODLE SOUP

INGREDIENTS

- 1 tablespoon canola oil
- 2 celery ribs, chopped
- 2 medium carrots, chopped
- 1 medium onion, chopped
- 8 cups reduced-sodium chicken broth
- 1/2 teaspoon dried basil
- 1/4 teaspoon pepper
- 3 cups uncooked whole-wheat egg noodles (about 4 ounces)
- 3 cups coarsely chopped rotisserie chicken
- 1 tablespoon minced fresh parsley

DIRECTIONS

- In a 6-qt. stockpot, heat oil over medium-high heat. Add celery, carrots and onion; cook and stir for 5-7 minutes or until tender.
- Add broth, basil and pepper; bring to a boil. Stir in noodles; cook for 12-14 minutes or until al dente. Stir in chicken and parsley; heat through.

MASHED POTATOES WITH CHEDDAR

INGREDIENTS

- 3 pounds potatoes, peeled and cubed (about 6 cups)
- 1 to 1-1/4 cups half-and-half cream
- 3 tablespoons butter
- 1 teaspoon salt
- 3 cups shredded extra-sharp cheddar cheese

DIRECTIONS

- Place potatoes in a 6-qt. stockpot; add water to cover. Bring to a boil. Reduce heat; cook, uncovered, 15-20 minutes or until tender. Meanwhile, in a small saucepan, heat cream, butter and salt until butter is melted, stirring occasionally.
- Drain potatoes; return to pot. Mash potatoes, gradually adding the cream mixture. Stir in cheese.
-

CHOCOLATE AVOCADO PUDDING

INGREDIENTS

- 2 large ripe avocados, peeled, pitted and cubed

- ½ cup cocoa powder
- ½ cup brown sugar
- ½ cup coconut milk
- 2 tsp vanilla extract
- 1 pinch ground cinnamon

DIRECTIONS

- Blend avocados, cocoa powder, brown sugar, coconut milk, vanilla extract, and cinnamon in a blender until smooth.
- Refrigerate pudding until chilled, approximately 30 minutes

APPLE CRUMBLE

INGREDIENTS

- 2 110g tubs unsweetened apple puree
- 1 tsp cinnamon
- ½ cup quick oats
- ¾ cup water
- Extra cinnamon and brown sugar

DIRECTIONS

1. Preheat the oven to 200°C.
2. Place oats and water in a microwave-safe bowl. Microwave on high for 1 minute.

Stir. Microwave again for 50 seconds. Remove from the microwave and cool. Transfer to a blender and blend for 1 minute on high or until smooth.

3. Place apple puree into 2 ramekins. Mix ½ tsp cinnamon into each ramekin.
4. Cover the apple with 2 tbsp oat mixture. Sprinkle with the desired amount of cinnamon and brown sugar.
5. Bake for 8–10 minutes.
6. Dust with cinnamon and brown sugar if desired then serve.

BAKED CUSTARD

INGREDIENTS

- 3 eggs
- 2 tbsp sugar
- 1 tsp vanilla
- 2½ cups of milk
- nutmeg or cinnamon

DIRECTIONS

1. Preheat the oven to 160°C (140°C fan-forced).
2. Beat eggs, sugar and vanilla together lightly.

3. Gently warm milk over the stove, before adding gradually to the egg mixture, stirring constantly.
4. Pour mixture into a shallow ovenproof dish, and sprinkle with nutmeg and/or cinnamon.
5. Place the dish in a water bath, with enough water to come halfway up the sides of the dish.
6. Bake in the oven for 30 minutes, before reducing the heat to 140°C (120°C fan-forced) for a further 20–30 minutes until set .

MAPLE SWEET CARROT PUREE

INGREDIENTS

- 5 cups fresh, canned, or frozen carrots
- 1/8th cup butter and ¼ cup maple syrup
- salt to taste

INSTRUCTIONS

1. Place carrots in 1 cup salted water, cover the pot and bring to a boil
2. Reduce heat to medium-low and simmer until fork tender (able to mash with tines of a fork)

3. Drain carrots
4. Blend warm carrots with butter and maple syrup until the texture is smooth

PUMPKIN BROWNIE PUREE

Ingredients:

- 1 box brownie mix
- ¼ cup pumpkin puree
- Milk, approximately 3 t per brownie

INSTRUCTIONS:

1. Preheat oven to 350 ° F
2. Grease 9×9 pan
3. In a bowl, mix the brownie mix and pumpkin puree until smooth
4. Spread into greased pan and bake 20-25 minutes
5. Allow brownies to cool
6. Place the desired amount of brownie into the blender. Add milk 1 t at a time and blend until a smooth texture is achieved.
7. If brownie becomes too runny, add a little bit more brownie and blend to thicken

MEAT LOAF PUREE

INGREDIENTS:

- 3 oz meatloaf
- 1 small boiled potato
- 1 small boiled carrot
- 2 tbsp brown gravy
- 1 cube beef bouillon

INSTRUCTIONS:

1. Cut meatloaf, potato, and carrots into cubes
2. Place all ingredients in a blender
3. Blend until smooth

BEVERAGES

CRUSHED ICE (IN A BLENDER)

Fill container with cold water to 2-cup level. Add ice cubes as needed to fill container to 4-cup level. Cover, CRUSH until ice is finely chopped. Pour into sieve immediately and drain. Use for making iced drinks, desserts, and chilling foods in a hurry.

INGREDIENTS

MOCHA FRAPP~

- 112 cup cold milk
- 2 tsps. instant coffee
- 1/8 tsp. cinnamon
- 1/2 pint chocolate or vanilla ice cream

INSTRUCTIONS

Blend.

ORANGE FRAPPE

INGREDIENTS

- 1 (6 oz.) can frozen orange juice concentrate, partially thawed
- 3 cups cracked ice
- 3 oz. bourbon, gin or vodka (optional)
- (Add a dash of bitters, if you like.)

INSTRUCTIONS

- In blender, GRIND all ingredients about 1 minute or until slushy.
- Mound in glasses and serve at once.

COTTAGE CHEESE COCKTAIL

INGREDIENTS

- 1 cup chilled grape juice
- 1/2 cup cottage cheese (cold)
- 2 tsps. sugar or honey

INSTRUCTION

Blend and drink.

FRUIT DRINK

INGREDIENTS

- 1 jar strained fruit
- 1/4 oz. juice

INSTRUCTIONS

- Blend.
- Use fruits and juices such as:
- Bananas, Oranges jc.
- Pears, Apple jc.
- Peaches, Orange jc.
- Pears, Pear Nectar

- Applesauce, Cranberry jc.
- Plums, Grape jc.
- Plums, Pineapple jc.
- Apricots, Pineapple jc.
- Applesauce, Apple jc.
- Apricots, Apricot Nectar
- Plums, Peach Nectar
- Peaches, Pineapple jc.
- Bananas, Pear Nectar
- Pears, Orange Jc

STRAWBERRY NECTAR

INGREDIENTS

- 1 cup sweet orange juice
- 3 tbsps. sugar
- 1 cup fresh strawberries
- 1 cup cracked ice

INSTRUCTIONS

Blend to desired consistency and muin.

VIRGIN PINA COLADA

INGREDIENTS

- 1-1/2 cups fresh pineapple
- 1/2 cup diluted apple juice
- 1 tsp. coconut extract
- 1/2 tsp. rum extract
- Sugar to taste
- 2-1/2 to 3 cups ice

INSTRUCTIONS

- Blend together pineapple, apple juice, extracts and sugar until smooth.
- Add ice and blend again until smooth and thick.

CHOCOLATE BANANA MALT

INGREDIENTS

- 1/2 cup Half & Half
- 1 tbsp. chocolate malted milk
- 1/2 cup ice cream
- 1 egg
- 1 ripe banana

Blend to desired consistency.

CUSTARD NOG

INGREDIENT

- 3/4 cup ice cream
- 2/3 cup eggnog

INSTRUCTIONS

Blend ingredients together.

CREAMY MILKSHAKE

INGREDIENTS

- 1/2 cup whipping cream
- 1/2 cup ice cream
- 2 tbsps. instant pudding mix (any flavor)
- 1 tbsp. sugar
- (For extra protein add 2 tbsps. dry protein powder.)

INSTRUCTIONS

Blend ingredients together.

EXTRA THICK MILKSHAKE

INGREDIENTS

- 1/4 cup ice cream
- 1/2-1 cup pudding

INSTRUCTIONS

Blend ingredients together.

SPECIAL "INSTANT BREAKFAST" SHAKE

INGREDIENTS

- 1 pkg. instant breakfast powder
- 8 oz. milk
- 2 tbsps. + 2 tsps. instant pudding mix

Blend ingredients together.

STRAWBERRYEBANANA MILKSHAKE

INGREDIENTS

- 2 cups milk
- 2 scoops vanilla ice cream
- 1 banana, peeled and sliced
- 1/2 cup fresh strawberries, hulled

In blender, LIQUEFY all ingredients 45 seconds. Strain. Pour into 2 tall

CHILLED GLASSES.

INGREDIENTS

THICK MOCHA SHAKE

- 2 cups chilled milk
- 1 pint chocolate ice cream, cubed
- 1/4 cup chocolate syrup
- 1 tbsp. instant coffee
- Whipped cream

In blender, BEAT all ingredients except whipped cream until well mixed,

about 10 seconds. Pour into 4 tall glasses. Top
with whipped cream.

APRICOT SMOOTHIE

INGREDIENTS

- 1/2 cup milk
- 2 jars strained apricots
- 1 cup vanilla ice cream

Blend.

BANANA SMOOTHIE

INGREDIENTS

- 1 cup cold milk
- 2 ripe bananas
- 1 cup cracked ice or 1 cup vanilla ice
  cream

Blend to desired consistency.

COFFEE SMOOTHIE

INGREDIENTS

- 1 tbsp. instant coffee
- 1-1/2 cups vanilla ice cream
- 1 tbsp, sugar

Blend.

DREAMSICLE SMOOTHIE

INGREDIENTS

- 1-1/2 cups fresh orange juice
- 1 ripe banana
- 1 tsp. vanilla
- Sugar to taste
- 2-1/2 to 3 cups ice

Blend together orange juice, banana, vanilla and sugar until smooth.

Add ice and blend again until smooth and thick.

MELON SMOOTHIE

INGREDIENTS

- 1/2 cup diluted apple juice (diluted in half)
- 1-1/2 cups fresh cantaloupe, peeled and cubed
- Sugar to taste
- 2-1/2 to 3 cups ice

Blend together apple juice, cantaloupe and sugar until smooth. Add ice and blend again until smooth and thick.

MINTED MELON SMOOTHIE

INGREDIENTS

- 1/2 cup diluted apple juice (diluted in half)
- 1-1/2 cups honeydew melon, peeled and cubed
- Few sprigs of fresh mint
- Sugar to taste
- 2-1/2 to 3 cups ice

- ❖ Blend together apple juice, honeydew

melon, mint and sugar until

❖ smooth. Add ice and blend again until smooth and thick.

PEACH SMOOTHIE

INGREDIENTS

- 1 cup canned peaches
- 2 cups ice cream - vanilla

Blend.

PINEAPPLE SMOOTHIE

- 1 cup canned crushed pineapple (blended and strained)
- 2 cups vanilla ice cream
- 2 drops peppermint extract

Blend.

YOGURT STRAWBERRY SMOOTHIE

INGREDIENTS

- 1 cup frozen strawberries with juice
- 1 cup yogurt (plain)
- Honey or sugar to taste

Blend and strain.

DESSERTS

LEMON CHEESE CAKE

INGREDIENTS

- 1/4 cup lemon juice
- 4 pkgs. (3 oz. each) cream cheese
- 2 eggs, beaten
- 3/4 cup granulated sugar

Combine lemon juice and cream cheese. Cream well. Add beaten eggs and sugar. Beat until fluffy. Bake at 350" for 15 to 20 minutes. Remove from oven; cool 5 minutes.

TOPPING

INGREDIENTS

- 1 tbsp. sugar
- 1 tbsp. grated lemon rind
- 1 cup sour cream

Mix together. Spread over pie. Return to oven and bake 10 minutes. Chill at least 5 hours before serving. Decorate top with lemon slices, if desired.

LEMONY LIGHT CHEESE CAKE

INGREDIENTS

- 2 envelopes unflavored gelatin
- 1/4 lemon (pulp only)
- 1/2 cup hot milk
- 2 egg yolks
- 1 (8 oz.) pkg. cream cheese, cubed and softened
- 1/2 cup heavy cream
- 1 cup cracked ice

In blender, grind gelatin, lemon and hot milk for 40 seconds. Add sugar, egg yolks and cream cheese. Mix 30 seconds. Scrape sides of container with rubber spatula. Mix 20 seconds adding cream and ice. Continue to push mixture to center. Pour into 9 inch layer cake pan. Chill until firm.

APPLE CUSTARD

INGREDIENTS

- 1/3 cup sugar
- 3/4 cup hot milk
- 1/3 cup diced cooked, peeled apple
- 1 tbsp. honey
- 1 egg

Blend all ingredients well and strain to remove apple pieces. Place in custard cups. Bake in a pan of hot water in 325" oven for 40 minutes, (or on a rack inside a saucepan making sure to add enough water to come 1 inch above rack. Cover and cook on top of stove 15 to 20 minutes over low heat making sure water boils slowly.)

Remove skin from top of custard and serve.

BAKED CARAMEL CUSTARD

INGREDIENTS

- 1 cup sugar
- 4 cups milk, scalded
- 6 eggs
- 2 tsps. vanilla
- 1/2 tsp. salt

Melt sugar in small heavy skillet over medium heat until it forms an amber-colored syrup. WHIP in blender scalded milk, eggs, vanilla and salt 10 seconds, adding sugar syrup through opening in top while motor is running. Pour into shallow 1-1/2 quart baking dish. Set baking dish in shallow pan on oven rack. Pour hot water into outer pan until 1 inch deep. Bake in moderate oven (350") 1 hour or until knife inserted in center comes out clean. Remove from water and cool on rack.

COTTAGE CHEESE CUSTARD

INGREDIENTS

- 3/4 cup hot milk
- 1/3 cup cottage cheese
- Dash nutmeg
- 1 tbsp. honey
- 1 egg

Blend all ingredients well. Divide into 3 custard cups. Bake in a pan of hot water in 325" oven, about 40 minutes, (or on a rack inside a saucepan making sure to add enough water to come 1 inch above rack.

Cover and cook on top of stove 15-20 minutes over low heat making sure water boils slowly).

Remove skin from top of custard and serve.

EGG CUSTARD

INGREDIENTS

- 4 eggs
- 1 cup sugar
- 1 tsp. nutmeg

- 1-1/2 cups milk
- Dash salt

Beat eggs; add sugar, nutmeg, milk, and salt. Mix and place in custard cups. Bake for 30 minutes at 350". (Place cups in pan of hot water).

PINEAPPLE RICE CUSTARD

INGREDIENTS

- 2/3 cup milk
- 1/2 cup cooked rice
- 1 egg
- 1/3 cup canned crushed pineapple

Blend all ingredients well and strain. Place in custard cups. Bake in a pan of hot water in 325" oven for 40 minutes (or on a rack inside a saucepan making sure to add enough water to come 1 inch above rack. Cover and cook on top of stove 15-20 minutes over low heat making sure water boils slowly).

Remove skin from top of custard and serve.

PUMPKIN CUSTARD

INGREDIENTS

- 1 1/2 cups cooked pumpkin (see note below)
- 2 large eggs
- 1 1/2 cups evaporated milk (or evaporated skim milk)
- 1/4 cup flour (or whole wheat flour)
- 1/2 cup sugar
- 1/2 tsp. ginger
- 1/2 tsp. cinnamon
- 1/2 tsp. nutmeg
- 1/4 tsp. cloves
- 1/4 tsp. salt
- 1/2 tsp. vanilla

(For pumpkin, you may substitute an equal amount of hubbard squash or

Pur6ed carrots. The squash makes a sweeter pie and sweetening may need to be adjusted to taste for different ingredients.)

Add well-beaten eggs to pumpkin; mix well. Stir in milk. Combine dry

Ingredients; add to mixture. Add vanilla. Spray custard cups with nonstick coating, pour in custard. Place cups in pan of hot water and bake at 350" for about 1 hour. Test with knife blade; cool on rack and do not serve until cooled to lukewarm.

LIME DIVINE

INGREDIENTS

- 21'3 cup boiling water
- 2 envelopes unflavored gelatin
- 1/2 cup sugar
- 1 (6 02.) can limeade or lemonade concentrate, thawed
- 2 heaping cups cracked ice

In blender, GRIND water and gelatin 60 seconds. Add sugar and GRIND 5 seconds. Add limeade and ice and SHRED 60 seconds or until ice is crushed. Let stand 1 minute. Spoon into serving dishes.

LIME-PEAR DESSERT

INGREDIENTS

- 1-1/2 quarts boiling water
- 12 oz. lime flavored gelatin
- 2 cans purEed pears
- Whipped topping

Add water to gelatin mix; stir until gelatin is dissolved. Stir in 2 cans Pur6ed pears. Portion into individual molds; chill until firm. Top each portion with whipped topping.

PEACH MELBA
Fill tart shells with pur6ed peaches. Spoon melted raspberry jelly over top. Chill; garnish with whipped topping.

APRICOT CHIFFON PIE

INGREDIENTS

- 2 eggs, separated

- 2 tbsps. sugar
- 2 envelopes unflavored gelatin
- 1/2 cup strained apricots
- 1/2 cup orange-juice concentrate or apricot nectar
- 1/2 cup hot milk
- 1/4 cup sugar
- 1 cup heavy cream
- 1 heaping cup cracked ice

Beat egg whites with electric or rotary beater until soft peaks form.

Gradually add the 2 tablespoons sugar and continue beating until stiff. In blender, GRIND gelatin, apricots, orange-juice concentrate or apricot nectar and hot milk 40 seconds. Add sugar and egg yolks and GRIND 15 seconds. 'Add cream and SHRED 40 seconds, gradually adding ice through opening in top while motor is running. Fold apricot mixture into beaten egg whites until smooth. Pour into chilled glasses. Chill until firm, at least 4 hours.

CHEESECAKE PIE

INGREDIENTS

- 2 (8 oz.) pkgs. cream cheese, cut up
- 2/3 cup sugar
- 3 eggs
- 1/4 tsp. almond extract
- 1 cup dairy sour cream
- 3 tbsps. sugar
- 1 tsp. vanilla

Beat together cream cheese, the 2/3 cup sugar, eggs, and almond extract.

Pour into an ungreased 9-inch pie plate. Bake in a 350" oven about 35 minutes.

In a small bowl stir together sour cream, the 3 tablespoons sugar, and vanilla; spread atop cheese mixture. Cool. Cover and chill at least 1 hour. Cut into wedges to serve.

CHOCOLATE CHIFFON PIE

INGREDIENTS

- 1 cup evaporated milk, chilled icy-cold

- 1 envelope unflavored gelatin
- 3/4 cup sugar
- 1/8 tsp. salt
- 1 egg yolk
- 3/4 cup milk
- 3 (1 oz.) squares unsweetened chocolate, cut in 4 pieces each
- 1 tsp. vanilla or mint flavoring

In blender, WHIP evaporated milk 60 seconds or until stiff, being careful not to overbeat. Empty into a bowl and chill while preparing filling.

BEAT all remaining ingredients, except vanilla, 20 seconds. Empty into saucepan and cook and stir over medium heat just until mixture begins to steam. Do not boil. Return to container and BLEND 40 seconds or until smooth. Pour into bowl and chill until mixture mounds when spooned. Fold in whipped milk and vanilla. Pour into parfait glasses and chill until firm. Garnish with whipped cream, if you wish.

FROZEN CRANBERRY VELVET PIE

INGREDIENTS

- 18-oz. pkg. cream cheese, softened

- 1 cup whipping cream
- 1/4 cup sugar
- 1/2 tsp. vanilla
- 1 (16 oz.) can cranberry sauce

Beat cream cheese until fluffy. Combine whipping cream, sugar and vanilla; whip until thickened but not stiff. Gradually add to the cream cheese, beating until smooth and creamy. Fold the cranberry sauce into the whipped mixture. Freeze until firm. Remove from freezer 10 to 15 minutes before serving. To serve, top with additional whipped cream.

EGG NOG PIE

INGREDIENTS

- 1 cup milk
- 1 pkg. instant vanilla pudding
- 1-1/2 tsps. rum flavoring
- 1 cup whipping cream

Whip the cream until stiff and refrigerate. Combine the pudding, milk and flavoring; beat until consistency of whipped cream, but do not overbeat. Combine with whipped cream, folding method. Refrigerate for 2 to 3 hours. Sprinkle the top of pie with nutmeg.

IMPOSSIBLE PIE

INGREDIENTS

- 4 eggs
- 1 stick butter
- 2 cups milk
- 1/2 cup sugar
- 1 tsp. coconut extract
- 1/2 cup Bisquick
- 1 tsp. vanilla

Put all the above in blender and blend for 2 minutes. Bake in 9" pie plate

that has been buttered and floured. Bake 45 minutes at 375". Chill for 3 hours.

KEY LIME PIE

Butter Crunch Crust:

- 1/2 cup butter
- 1/4 cup brown sugar, packed
- 1 cup flour, sifted

Combine all ingredients and mix well. Spread in a 13x9" pan and bake at 400" for 12 to 15 minutes until golden. Stir immediately and press into a 9" pie pan and cool.

Filling:

- 1 can Eagle Brand sweetened condensed milk
- 4 egg yolks
- 1/2 cup key lime juice or 114 cup lime and 112 cup lemon juice
- 1 large egg white, beaten stiff

Combine milk, egg yolks and juice; fold in beaten egg white. Pour into crust.

Meringue:

- 3 egg whites
- 6 tbsps. sugar
- 1/2 tsp. cream of tartar

Beat egg whites; gradually add sugar and cream of tartar and beat until stiff and glossy. Cover filling with meringue. Bake pie at 350" until

VEGETABLES

CONGEALED AVOCADO SALAD

INGREDIENTS

- 1 (3 oz.) pkg. lime-flavored gelatin
- 1 cup boiling water
- 1 (3 oz.) pkg. cream cheese
- 1 avocado, mashed
- 1 small onion, chopped very fine
- 118 tsp. celery salt
- 1 pimiento, mashed
- 1/2 cup mayonnaise

Combine together and chill.

BAKED BEANS

Buy a can or jar of your favorite baked beans. Blend them with bean liquid or water.

Optional: add a drop or two of Liquid Smoke or cooked onions.

MEXICAN REFRIED BEANS

INGREDIENTS

- 1 can refried beans

Add water or chicken soup to blend to right consistency. Can add bacon drippings for more flavor.

SWEDISH BAKED BEANS

INGREDIENTS

- 3/4 cup catsup or chili sauce
- 1/2 medium onion, finely chopped
- 1 medium apple, peeled, cored, and cut into I-inch chunks
- 1/3 cup well-drained sweet pickle relish
- 1 tbsp. brown sugar
- 1 tsp. prepared mustard
- 2 cans (1 lb. 4 oz.) pork and beans

Combine catsup or chili sauce and onion in blender container. BLEND until onion is chopped, about 30 seconds. Stop motor as needed and push ingredients into blades with rubber spatula. Add apple chunks, 1/2 at a time; BLEND until chopped, 20 to 25 seconds. Pour into covered frypan. Add remaining ingredients; mix. Bring to simmering stage; cover and cook slowly until heated and flavors are well blended, 25 to 30 minutes, stirring frequently.

CARROT CUSTARD

INGREDIENTS

- 2 cups cooked sliced carrots
- 3 eggs
- 1/4 cup milk
- 1 small onion halved and chopped
- 3 tbsps. melted butter
- 2 tbsps. flour
- 1 1/2 tsps. salt
- 1/4 tsp. pepper

Put in blender and blend for 10 seconds. Turn into 6 buttered 5 02. custard cups, place in pan with 1 " hot water. Bake in pre-heated oven at 350" for 45 minutes. Unmold and garnish.

CARROT ORANGE PURBE

INGREDIENTS

- 4 Ibs. carrots, peeled and cut into l-inch rounds
- 8 tbsps. unsalted butter
- 1-1/2 cups warmed chicken broth
- 1/2 cup fresh orange juice
- 2-1/2 tsps. ground cardamon
- 1-1/2 tsps. salt
- 1/4 tsp. cayenne pepper

Place carrots in a large pot. Cover with water and bring to a boil. Cook for 30 minutes, or until carrots are very tender.

Drain carrots and place in large bowl. Add remaining ingredients - mix well.

In a food processor fitted with a steel blade, process mixture in small batches until smooth. Remove to a bowl as processed.

To reheat, return puree to a saucepan over low heat; stir well until heated through. Or transfer to an ovenproof serving dish covered with foil; heat in a preheated 350" F oven for 25 minutes, or until steaming hot.

CARROT PUDDING

INGREDIENTS

- 1 cup carrots, grated
- 1 cup potatoes, grated
- 1 cup flour
- 1 cup sugar
- 2 tbsps. butter, melted
- 1/2 tsp. soda
- 1/2 tsp. salt
- 1/2 tsp. cloves
- 1/2 tsp. cinnamon
- 1/2 tsp. nutmeg
- 1/2 tsp. vanilla

Mix all ingredients and cook in double boiler until pudding consistency.

Serve either warm or cold with Brown Sauce (Recipe below).

BROWN SAUCE FOR CARROT PUDDING

INGREDIENTS

- 1 cup brown sugar
- 2 tbsps. flour
- 1 cup boiling water
- 1 tbsp. butter
- Bourbon or rum
- Vanilla, if desired
- flavoring as desired

Mix flour and sugar; add boiling water and cook until thickened. Remove, cool, add flavoring.

CARROTS WITH A TWIST

Steam carrots until soft and tender. Blend in blender with melted butter until smooth. Strain. Add dash of orange liqueur. Place mixture in pastry tube and squeeze onto plate in an attractive manner.

EGGPLANT CASSEROLE

INGREDIENTS

- 1 small green pepper, chopped and blended
- 2 tsps. onion powder
- 1/4 cup margarine
- 1 to 1-1/2 *eggplant peeled, sliced, cooked and mashed
- 2 eggs, beaten
- 1 cup homogenized milk
- 2 tbsps. chopped pimiento, blended
- 1/2 tsp. salt
- 1/8 tsp. pepper
- 1 cup cracker crumbs . soaked in milk
- 6 oz. American cheese, grated

Preheat oven to 350". Saute pureed green pepper in margarine. Add onion powder. Combine with eggplant, egg, milk and crackers, pimiento, salt, pepper, and cheese. Pour into a greased casserole. Additional grated Cheese can be added on top. Bake 30-40 minutes.

*Eggplant needs to be young and tender. Soak slices in strong salt water

to eliminate bitter taste. Rinse before cooking.

PUR~ED PEAS

INGREDIENTS

- 4 cups raw fresh peas
- 3 tbsps. butter
- Salt and pepper

Boil the peas in as little water as possible until they are just done. Drain and pour into a blender. Run until you have a smooth puree. Scrape this puree into the top part of a double boiler (over boiling water), add the butter, salt, and pepper, and heat until the butter is melted and well combined with the peas.

GRATED POTATO CASSEROLE

INGREDIENTS

- 1 cup milk
- 3 eggs
- 1-1/2 tsps. salt
- 1/8 tsp. pepper
- 1 cup cubed cheddar cheese
- 2 tbsps. soft butter
- 1 small onion, quartered
- 4 medium potatoes, pared and cubed

Preheat oven to 350". Grease 1-1/2 quart casserole. Put all ingredients in blender in order listed. Cover and run on high just until all potatoes go through the blades. Pour into casserole and bake 1 hour.

POTATO GOURMET

INGREDIENTS

- 1 pck. Ore-Ida Potatoes O'Brien
- 1 pint sour cream
- 1 can Cream of Chicken Soup
- 10 oz. sharp cheddar cheese, grated
- 114 stick melted margarine

Mix all ingredients and bake 1 hour at 325"

POTATO NESTS

- 1 lb. creamed potatoes
- 4 eggs
- Seasoning
- 1 oz. grated cheese

Pipe a border of creamed potato around 4 scallop shells or dishes (or put the potato into a greased heat-proof dish and make 4 wells in it). Break an egg into each dish (or well) and sprinkle with salt, pepper and grated cheese. Bake in a moderate oven (350") until the eggs are set - about 10 to 15 minutes.

BAKED SWEET POTATOES

Scrub sweet potatoes. Bake at 375" to 400" for 40 to 45 minutes. Add butter, salt, and pepper to taste.

BLENDED SWEET POTATOES

INGREDIENTS

- 1/2 cup milk or chicken soup - or non-dairy creamer
- 1 egg
- 1/4 cup soft butter
- 3/4 cup brown sugar
- 1/2 tsp. salt, ginger, cinnamon
- 3 cups cooked sweet potato or 1 large can

Put ingredients in blender and blend well. Heat a few minutes until egg cooks. Strain if needed.

MASHED SWEET POTATOES

Peel hot cooked sweet potatoes. Mash. Beat until fluffy gradually adding hot milk as needed. Beat in salt, pepper, and butter to taste.

SWEET POTATO SOUFFL~

INGREDIENTS

- 6 egg yolks
- 3 cups cooked sweet potatoes (yams)
- 1/2 cup table cream
- 1 cup milk
- 1/2 tsp. salt
- 1 cup butter
- 1 tsp. vanilla
- 1 tsp. cinnamon
- 6 egg whites (stiffly beaten)

Whip egg yolks and sweet potatoes until well blended. Add cream, milk, salt, butter, vanilla and cinnamon, beating at high speed for 1 minute. Fold in egg whites and pour into baking dish. Bake at 375" for 45 minutes.

Variations: Try, 3 cups of cooked carrots, butternut or acorn squash, pumpkin or strained cream corn (may use small jars of Hines or Gerber strained corn to equal 3 cups).

RICOTTA SPINACH BAKE

INGREDIENTS

- 1 bunch fresh spinach or 1 10-oz. pkg. frozen spinach
- 1 cup Ricotta cheese
- Nutmeg, grated
- 1 cup Parmesan cheese, grated
- 4 eggs, lightly beaten
- Salt and pepper

Wash spinach and cook for a few minutes. Squeeze out all liquid and chop: should be about 3/4 cup. Combine spinach with Ricotta, a little nutmeg and 1/2 cup of Parmesan cheese. Pour over the bottom. Combine eggs with cream, milk, salt and pepper. Pour over Ricottaspinach mixture. Sprinkle with remaining Parmesan and bake at 375" for 30 minutes, or until a knife inserted in the center comes out clean. Let sit 10 minutes before serving.

SPINACH SOUFFLE

INGREDIENTS

- 2 tbsps. mayonnaise
- 2 tbsps. flour
- 1/2 cup milk
- 112 10 oz. pkg. frozen spinach, chopped, cooked and drained
- 114 tsp. onion powder
- 1/4 tsp. nutmeg
- Black pepper to taste
- 6 egg whites
- 3 tbsps. Parmesan cheese

In small heavy saucepan, melt margarine. Blend in flour. Cook until mixture is smooth and bubbly. Remove from heat and gradually stir in milk.

Return to heat and bring mixture to a boil, stirring constantly. Cook 1 minute. Remove from heat, stir in spinach, onion powder, nutmeg and

Pepper. Beat egg whites until stiff, fold gently into spinach mixture. Sprinkle with Parmesan. Pour into 1 3/4 quart casserole. Bake at 350" for 35 minutes.

SOUPS

CRAB BISQUE

INGREDIENTS

- 2-112 cups milk
- 1 tbsp. flour
- 1 tbsp. butter
- 1 tsp. celery salt
- Dash pepper
- 2/3 cup crab meat (carefully remove all cartilage)
- 1 drop tabasco

Place milk, flour, butter, salt, pepper, and tabasco in blender. Blend well.

Add crab meat. Blend. Pour in saucepan - boil over low heat. Stir constantly until done. Strain and serve.

CURRIED FISH BISQUE

INGREDIENTS

- 2-1/2 cups milk
- 1 tbsp. flour
- 1 tbsp. butter
- 1 tsp. salt
- 1/4 tsp. curry
- Dash paprika
- Dash pepper
- 2/3 or 1 cup cooked lean white meat fish (NO BONES)

Place milk, flour, butter, salt, curry, paprika, and pepper in blender. Blend well. Add fish. Blend. Pour in saucepan. Boil over low heat. Stir

constantly until done. Strain and serve.

LOBSTER BISQUE

INGREDIENTS

- 2-1/2 cups milk
- 1 tbsp. flour

- 1 tbsp. butter
- 1 tsp. salt
- 1/8 tsp. celery salt
- 1/4 tsp. paprika
- Dash pepper
- 2/3 cup cooked lobster meat (1 small South African Rock Lobster tail or
- 1 can lobster meat)

Place milk, flour, butter, salt, celery salt, paprika, and pepper in blender. Blend. Add lobster meat. Blend well. Pour in saucepan and boil over low heat. Stir constantly until done. Strain and serve.

SALMON BISQUE

INGREDIENTS

- 2-1/2 cups milk
- 1 tbsp. flour
- 1 tbsp. butter
- 1 tsp. salt
- Dash pepper
- 1/2 cup cooked salmon or .1 small can of salmon (NO BONES)

Blend salmon and set aside. Place milk, flour, butter, salt, and pepper in blender. Blend well. Add salmon. Blend. Pour in saucepan and boil over low heat. Stir constantly until done. Strain and serve.

BASIC SEAFOOD BISQUE

INGREDIENTS

- 2-1/2 cups milk
- 1 tbsp. flour
- 1 tbsp. butter
- 1 tsp. salt
- Dash pepper
- 2/3 cups cooked (with special seasoning) or canned seafood

Place milk, flour, butter, salt and pepper in blender. Blend well - add seafood - blend. Pour in saucepan and boil on low heat. Stir constantly until done. Strain and serve.

SHRIMP BISQUE c COLD

INGREDIENTS

- 2 cups plain yogurt or non-dairy creamer
- 1/2 tsp. prepared mustard
- 1/2 tsp. salt
- 1/2 tsp. sugar
- 1 can shrimp
- 1/2 cup diced, peeled cucumber

Put everything in blender. Blend well. Strain. Chill before serving.

TUNA CHOWDER

INGREDIENTS

- 1/4 tsp. onion powder
- 2 tbsps. melted margarine
- 1 can cream of celery soup (10-112 oz.)
- 1 can cream of mushroom soup

Blend all ingredients in blender. Put through strainer to remove larger pieces. Garnish with paprika. Heat. (If too salty, try salt-free tuna or saltfree soups).

CHICKEN AVOCADO SOUP COLD

INGREDIENTS

- 2-1/2 cups chicken broth
- 2 cups sliced avocado
- 1 tsp. salt
- Pepper (optional)
- 2 tbsps. sherry
- 1/4 cup whipping cream or non-dairy creamer (optional)

Put everything in blender. Cover and blend well. Chill.

CHICKEN BISQUE

INGREDIENTS

- 1 cup chicken broth
- 1 tbsp. flour
- 3 tbsps. butter

- 1/2 tsp. salt
- Dash pepper
- 118 tsp. curry powder
- 1 spray celery leaves
- 314 cup diced cooked chicken
- or 112 cup strained chicken
- 1 cup light cream or Half & Half

Blend broth, flour, butter, seasonings, celery leaves, and chicken. Strain Pour in saucepan and add cream. Heat thoroughly to just a boil.

CURRIED CHICKEN SOUP

INGREDIENTS

- 114 tsp. onion powder
- 114 tsp. celery salt
- 118 tsp. curry powder
- 1 tbsp. butter or margarine
- 1 can condensed cream of chicken soup (10-1/2 02.)
- 112 soup can milk
- 112 cup cooked chicken, blended

Blend all ingredients in blender. Put through strainer to remove larger pieces. Heat. All people smile in the same language.

YOGURT BORSCHT COLD

INGREDIENTS

- 1 cup plain yogurt
- 3/4 cup sour cream
- 1/4 tsp. salt
- 1/4 tsp. celery salt
- 1/4 tsp. onion salt
- 1 cup diced, cooked beets
- Sour cream for garnish

Add all ingredients in blender except for the sour cream for garnish. Blend until smooth. Chill. Serve with a spoonful of sour cream.

BROCCOLI CHOWDER

INGREDIENTS

- 1 10 oz. pkg. frozen broccoli

- 2 tsps. instant minced onion
- 1/2 cup boiling, salted water
- 2 cups milk
- 1 can condensed cream of potato soup
- 1/2 cup shredded Swiss cheese (2 oz.)

Cook broccoli and onion in the boiling salted water until tender. Do not drain. Stir in milk and soup, heat thoroughly. Add cheese, stirring until melted. Cool slightly. Place half at a time in blender. Blend until smooth. Serve chilled or hot.

CARROT VICHYSSOISE COLD

INGREDIENTS

- 2 tbsps. butter
- 2 scallions
- 2 cups chicken broth
- 2 cups diced, cooked carrots

Melt butter in small saucepan. Add sliced scallions and cook over moderate heat - about 5 minutes. Add 1 cup of the broth and cooked carrots, and bring to a boil. Cover and let simmer over low heat for 15 minutes. Place in blender and add the other cup of broth. Blend until smooth. Add cream and chill.

CAULIFLOWER SOUP

INGREDIENTS

- 1/4 cup chopped onion
- 4 tbsps. butter, melted
- 4 tbsps. flour
- 1 small cauliflower, cooked and pureed
- 2 cups milk
- 1 tsp. salt
- 1 egg yolk
- 2 tbsps. grated cheddar cheese
- 1/2 cup cooked and crumbled spicy sausage

Saute onion in butter until transparent. Add flour and stir until mixture thickens. Whisk incauliflower and milk. Heat, but do not boil. Whip in and mixture in blender. Blend well. Strain if necessary. salt, egg yolk, and cheese, stirring until slightly thickened. Put sausage

THICKENED STRAINED CREAM SOUP

INGREDIENTS

- 1/4 cup strained cream soup
- 1/4 cup smooth mashed potatoes

Combine soup and mashed potatoes. Mix well. Strain if necessary to remove lumps.

CUCUMBER VICHYSSOISE COLD

INGREDIENTS

- 1/4 cup sliced onion
- 2 cups diced cucumber, peeled
- 1/4 cup diced potatoes, raw
- 2 cups chicken broth
- 2 sprigs parsley
- 1/2 tsp. salt
- 1/8 tsp. pepper

- 1/4 tsp. dry mustard
- 1 cup heavy cream or evaporated milk

Put onion, cucumber, and potatoes in saucepan. Add chicken broth, parsley and seasonings. Bring to boil. Cover and cook until potatoes are tender. Pour off 1 cup of broth and set aside. Put cooked vegetables in blender. Cover and blend.wel1. Stir in 1 cup broth. Add more seasoning if you like. Strain well. Chill. Add cold milk or cream when you are ready to serve.

CURRIED LEEK SOUP COLD

INGREDIENTS

- 3 tbsps. butter or margarine
- 1 leek or 6 scallions - sliced
- 1 cup milk
- 1/2 tsp. salt
- 1/2 tsp. curry powder
- 1 cup light cream

Mashed potatoes to thicken

Melt butter in saucepan. Add leeks or scallions. Cook on moderate heat for 5 to 10 minutes, stirring often. Cool. Place in blender with milk and cream, salt or curry. Strain and chill. Add blended mashed potatoes to thicken.

CREAM OF MUSHROOM SOUP

INGREDIENTS

- 2-1/2 cups milk
- 1 tbsp. flour
- 2 tbsps. butter 5 minutes)
- 1 tsp. salt
- Dash pepper

Blend milk, flour, butter, salt, and pepper. Add mushrooms and onions. Blend. Pour into saucepan. Boil over low heat until mushrooms are tender, stirring frequently. Strain and serve.

MUSHROOM VELVET SOUP

INGREDIENTS

- 1-1/2 cups water

- 1 pkg. noodle soup mix
- 1/8 tsp. celery salt
- 1 slice of onion finely chopped or (1/8 tsp. onion powder)
- 3 tbsps. butter
- 1/4 to 1/2 lb. chopped mushrooms, cooked (not canned)
- 1 cup milk

Add 1-112 cups water to noodle soup mix, then add celery salt, onion, and butter. Cook for seven minutes. Blend. Add cooked mushrooms.

Blend well. Pour milk into saucepan, add blended mixture and heat. For variation; 1) add one cup strained vegetables - such as asparagus, beets, peas, spinach; 2) use 2/3 cup of blended strained seafood in place of mushrooms; or 3) try fresh basil and a little garlic juice. Be sure to strain well.

VICHYSSOISE ORIENTAL COLD

INGREDIENTS

- 1 cup diced potatoes

- 1/2 cup diced onions
- 1 cup diced, peeled apple
- 1/2 cup sliced tender celery (remove strings)
- 1 banana - sliced
- 1-1/2 cups chicken broth
- 1 tbsp. butter
- 1/2 tsp. curry powder
- 1 cup heavy cream
- 1/2 tsp. salt

Put vegetables, banana, apple, and broth in saucepan and bring to a boil.

Simmer over low heat until vegetables are tender. Pour slowly into blender and add salt, butter, and curry powder. Blend until smooth.

Strain. Let mixture cool. Stir cream into cooled mixture and chill.

FRESH PEA SOUP

INGREDIENTS

- 1 cup fresh or frozen green peas

- 1 tbsp. diced onion
- Dash pepper
- Dash ginger
- 2-1/2 cups chicken broth
- 1 tbsp. butter
- 2 tsps. flour or arrowroot

Combine peas, onions, and chicken broth. Cook until tender. Add pepper, ginger, and butter. Put everything into blender. Cover and blend well. Strain. Pour into saucepan, add flour or arrowroot to thicken, and bring to a boil stirring constantly. Simmer 5 minutes.

GREEN POTAGE

INGREDIENTS

- 1/3 cup butter
- 1/4 cup sliced scallions
- 2 cups raw or cooked potatoes
- 1 tsp. salt
- 2 cups chicken broth
- 1/2 bunch watercress
- 1 cup spinach leaves or 1 pkg. of frozen

chopped spinach
- 2 cups lettuce
-

Cook butter and scallions together for about 5 minutes over moderate heat. Stir often. Add potatoes, salt, and chicken broth. Bring to boil and cook covered for 10 minutes. Add coarsely cut watercress, spinach, and lettuce. Cook until vegetables are tender. Strain 1 cup of broth. Put

Vegetables and remaining broth in blender. Blend until smooth. Combine with reserved broth - stir. Strain. Add a dollop of sour cream and paprika at serving time.

CREAM OF POTATO SOUP

INGREDIENTS

- 1 cup diced, hot, cooked potatoes
- 2 cups milk - for richer soup use Half &a Half
- 2 tbsps. chopped onion
- 1 chicken bouillon cube and 1 tbsp. bouillon granules
- 1/2 tsp. salt

- Dash pepper
- 2 tbsps. butter

Place all ingredients in blender. Cover and blend until smooth. Pour into saucepan and heat thoroughly over moderate heat. Strain and serve.

SWEET POTATO SOUP

INGREDIENTS

- 1-1/2 cups diced or mashed cooked sweet potatoes
- 1 tbsp. butter
- 1 tbsp. flour
- 1-1/2 tsps. salt
- 1/4 tsp. ginger
- 1/8 tsp. cinnamon
- 1/8 tsp. nutmeg
- 1 tbsp. brown sugar
- 1 tsp. chicken broth or water
- 1 cup milk

Put everything except milk into blender. Blend well. Add milk. Cook stirring constantly until soup comes to a boil. Simmer over a low heat for 5 minutes. Serve immediately.

VEGETABLE BISQUE

INGREDIENTS

- 1-1/2 cups milk 3 tbsps. butter
- 1 beef or chicken bouillon cube 1/2 tsp. salt
- 1 cup water Dash pepper
- 2 tbsps. flour 1/8 tsp. oregano
- 1 cup cooked vegetables (any kind)

Blend all ingredients. Cook in saucepan until done. Strain.

BASIC CREAM OF VEGETABLE SOUP

INGREDIENTS

- 2-1/2 cups milk
- 1 tbsp. flour
- 2 tbsps. butter
- 1 tsp. salt
- Dash pepper
- 1 cup raw or cooked vegetables - or 1 pkg.

frozen chopped spinach and
Seasonings

- Mashed potatoes to thicken

Blend milk, flour, butter, salt, and pepper. Add vegetables and seasoning.

Blend well. Pour in saucepan. Boil over low heat stirring constantly. Add mashed potatoes to thicken. Strain and serve.

PERFECTION VEGETABLE SOUP

INGREDIENTS

- 1 cup water
- 2 beef bouillon cubes
- 1/4 cup diced onion
- 1/2 cup diced tender celery
- 1/2 cup sliced carrot
- 1 spray parsley
- 1 cooked potato
-

Place all ingredients in blender. Cover. Blend well. Pour into saucepan and bring to a boil.

Simmer over low heat for about 10 minutes.
Strain. Serve hot.

VEGETABLE VICHYSSOISE COLD

INGREDIENTS

- 1 cup diced cooked potatoes
- 1/4 cup sliced onions or scallions
- 1-1/2 cups chicken broth
- 1 cup raw green peas
- 1/8 tsp. celery salt
- 1/8 tsp. curry powder
- 1 cup heavy cream (1 small carton whip cream or non-dairy creamer)

Add potatoes, onions, broth, and peas in saucepan. Cook until onions and peas are tender. Place in blender (except cream) with seasonings.

Blend well. Strain. Combine with cream and chill.

SAUCES

ALFREDO SAUCE

INGREDIENTS

- 1 stick butter or margarine Garlic powder,
- liquid, or 1 clove of garlic pureed
- 1 small carton whipping cream
- 1/2 small carton sour cream
- Salt and pepper to taste Grated Parmesan cheese - 112 cup

Melt butter, add garlic on low heat, and both creams. Mix well and add salt and pepper if desired. Take from heat and add Parmesan cheese.

Blend.

Use over blended meats, vegetables, mashed potatoes, or blended pasta.

HERBED LEMON BUTTER SAUCE

INGREDIENTS

- 1/4 cup melted butter
- 2 tbsps. lemon juice
- 2 tbsps. finely chopped parsley
- 1/4 tsp. dill, rosemary or marjoram, crumbled
- 114 tsp. salt
- 1/8 tsp. coarsely ground pepper

Strain. Use for basting fish.

MUSHROOM BUTTER SAUCE

INGREDIENTS

Saute:

- 1 lb. chopped mushrooms
- 1 chopped onion
- 1/2 stick butter
- 1 tbsp. flour Salt and pepper

Blend all ingredients and strain.

Use over blended meats, vegetables, mashed potatoes, or blended pasta.

QUICK HERBED HOLLANDAISE SAUCE

INGREDIENTS

- I/2 cup butter
- 1-1/2 tbsps. fresh lemon juice
- 1/4 tsp. dill
- Generous dash white pepper
- 3 egg yolks, well-drained of whites
- 1 tbsp. finely chopped fresh parsley

In small saucepan, heat butter with lemon juice, choice of herbs and pepper until bubbly. Add slowly to egg yolks, beating constantly with wire whisk. Stir in parsley. Strain.

ZESTY SALMON SAUCE

INGREDIENTS

- 11'2 cup butter
- 3 tbsps. soy sauce
- 2 tbsps. catsup
- 1 tbsp. each Worcestershire sauce and dry

mustard

- 1 clove garlic, crushed

Combine ingredients in small saucepan; heat gently but thoroughly.

CONCLUTION

Eating and feeding tips

Always eat in smaller bites and chew food thoroughly. Special thickening powder might need to be added to drinks since watery liquids can be difficult to swallow.

Sitting upright while eating will reduce the risk of choking. Patients can also learn to tilt the head to make swallowing easier. These techniques reduce the risk of liquid getting into the airway (aspiration).

Clearing the throat with a little cough if liquid or a small piece of food gets stuck

Printed in Great Britain
by Amazon

22974492R00057